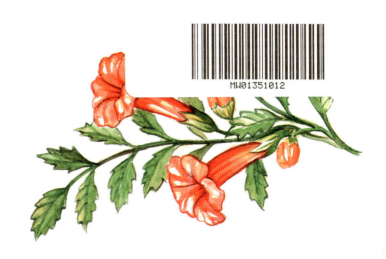

Color Me Calm

Stress Management Through Coloring

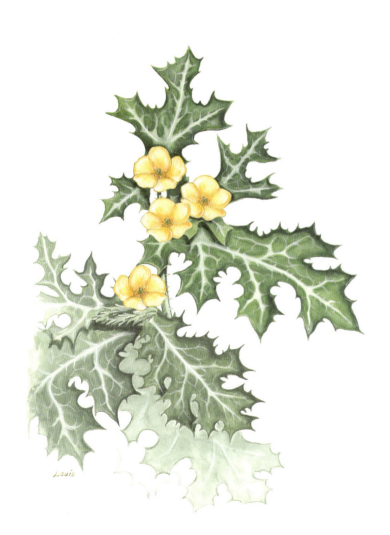

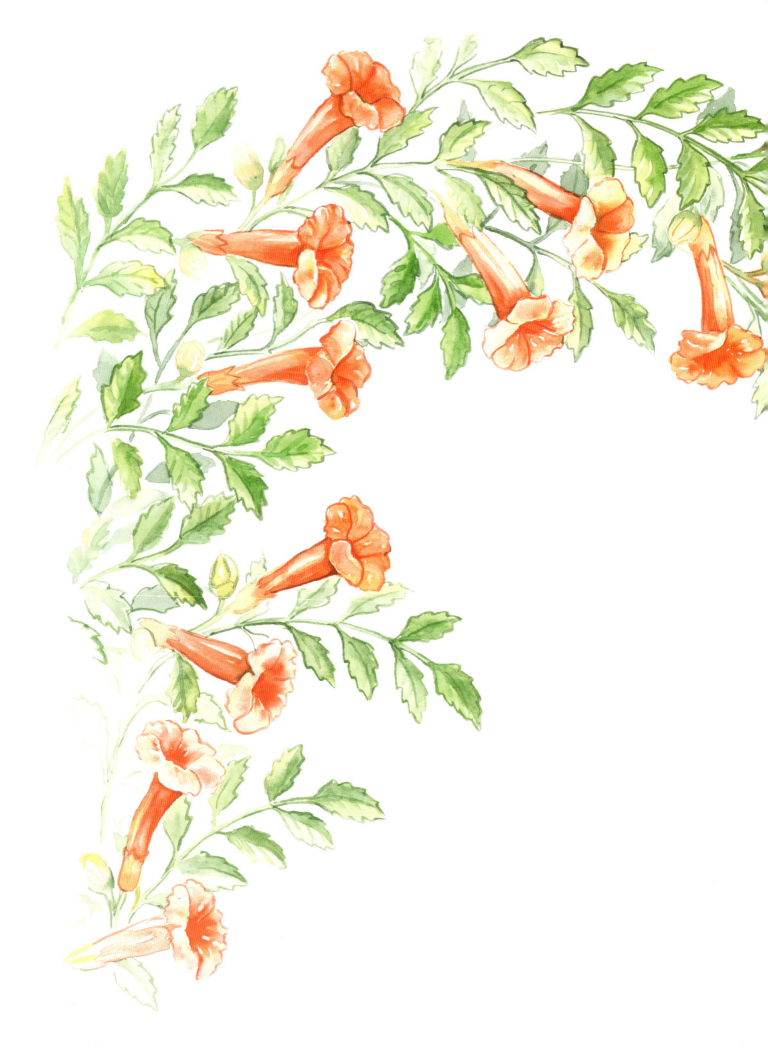

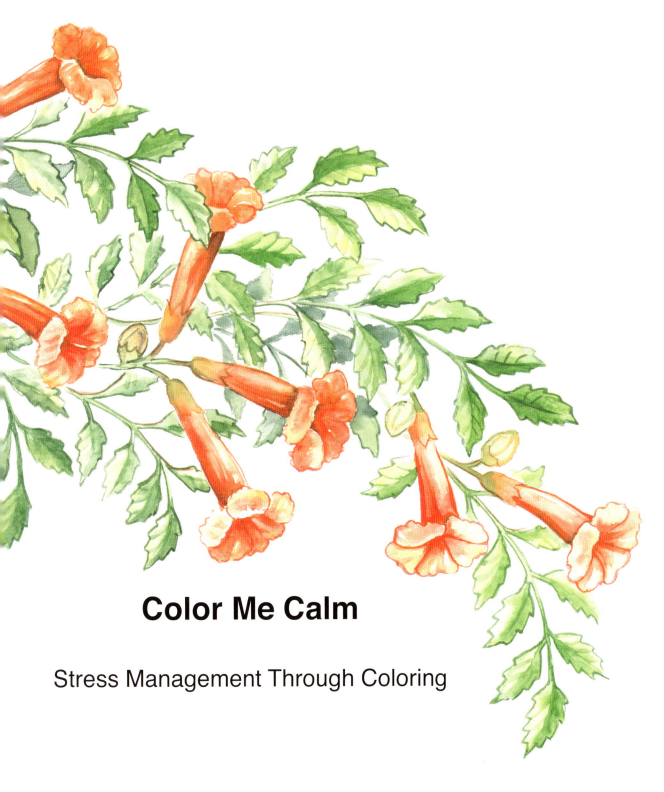

Color Me Calm

Stress Management Through Coloring

Featuring Florida Native Plants

Mary Virginia Graham and Madge Cloud

Illustrated by Louis Clark

This book is for our grandchildren, who remind us every day of the importance of wonder, joy, and play in our lives.

Copyright 2010 by Mary Virginia Graham and Madge Cloud
All rights reserved. No part of this book may be reproduced in any form or by any means, electronic or mechanical, including photocopying, microfilm, retrieval system, or any other information storage system without prior permission in writing from the authors.

Cover Art by Louis Clark

Every effort has been made to ensure accuracy of text, illustrations, and credits. Publisher assumes no liability for errors or omissions.

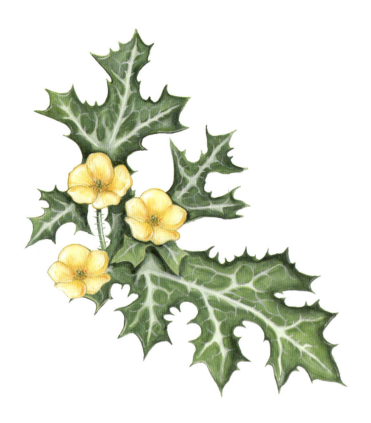

ISBN 978-0-615-36144-4

Publishing by
Color Me Calm
Gainesville, FL

Welcome to the *Color Me Calm* Coloring Book Series

The *Color Me Calm* series gives people of all ages an opportunity to experience the fun and relaxation of coloring. Books in the series have a common theme: They are all based on the assumption that positive affect or mood is inextricably linked to health — the well-being of one is intertwined with that of the other. A further assumption is that coloring, like other forms of art, is a technique with the potential to enhance physical, mental, and emotional health.

This first book focuses on the role of stress and stress management on mood. Future books will consider the benefits of a life spent practicing gratitude, mindfulness, spirituality, and other disciplines designed to help us down the path to a more joyful life. Plans for the coloring topics in forthcoming books include vintage quilt patterns, state birds, and Victorian dress.

We chose to feature native plants of Florida for you to color in this first book. Most, if not all, of the native plants included here are also native to other states. Many plants that flourish in Florida thrive elsewhere. What better way to discover the attraction of native plants than to color them, and watch them come alive. We hope that this experience leads you to visit a botanical garden in your area, or to make a decision to grow plants native to *your* state in your own backyard.

Acknowledgments

We would like to thank Sharren Gibbs for her creative presentation of the text for the book. Her gifts for quality and accuracy were indispensable in the production of this book. Also, a special thanks to Melani Jayne Graham, a talented 16 year-old junior at Gibbs High School, Pinellas County Center for the Arts, St. Petersburg, FL, who created the wonderful illustrations for the *Introduction*. And to Graham Holt Hardcastle, now 10 and in the 4th grade at Oak Hall School, Gainesville, FL, who, at age 6, drew the flowers on the last page of the book.

Sources for the plant descriptions used in this book are listed at the end of the book, on the *About the Authors* page.

Introduction

"Grandma, will you color with me?" asked my six-year-old grandson.

"Honey, I haven't colored since I was a little girl, and I wasn't that great at it even then!"

"Please, I found the perfect picture for you. Please! Please!"

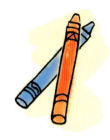

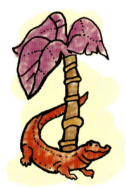

Who could resist that offer? So I sat down next to him, and within three minutes, I was chuckling to myself as I colored purple leaves on a palm tree and made a red alligator underneath it. We both laughed ourselves silly over that one! I hadn't felt so at peace, so relaxed, so joyous in, well, way too long.

A few days later, I talked about the "coloring experience," with my sister, Madge, during one of our frequent telephone conversations. I live in Florida and she lives near Chicago. She laughingly admitted that she herself had recently rediscovered the joys of coloring thanks to her youngest grandchild, Julia, also six at the time. We both agreed that we would like to bottle the pleasant feeling we had when we were coloring.

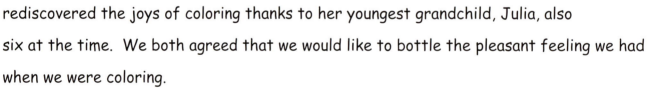

Bottling joy seemed a bit out of our reach, however, and being the pragmatic Southern women that we are, we quickly figured out another way to share our coloring epiphany. On that day, the idea was born for *Color Me Calm*, a coloring book that focuses on ways to make happiness happen by affirming positive affect or mood.

Over time, we have come to believe that the simple act of coloring may be a way for us to grow our creativity and de-stress our lives. But first, we must be willing to make time for ourselves and relinquish the mental space to spend time coloring. We think of the handyman one of us consulted recently about building additional shelving for storage in a bathroom. After spending several minutes gazing at all the stuff in the small room, he turned, and with a troubled look on his face, gravely asked, "Have you ever thought about de-cluttering?" Coloring is a way of mental de-cluttering.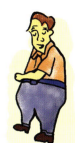

What we are suggesting to you is something that you already know how to do — something you already have warm feelings about, and something that can help you relax, de-stress, and, in fact, help you build a more joyous you: coloring.

Coloring coaxes us to change our point of view and calms our minds, giving our thoughts space to wander aimlessly. A rested mind takes us places we would otherwise have missed, and such mental meanderings are more likely to produce those eureka moments that can help us solve the problems of everyday life. Those tales about Sir Isaac Newton formulating the laws of gravity while lounging under a tree may be true!

Come along with us — spend a few minutes learning more about the role of stress in your life and ways in which coloring can help to reduce and manage stress. And, while you are expanding your horizons by trying something new, you can also learn a little about some of the wonderful native plants of Florida. We will guide you on a path that may enable you to be more creative, thoughtful, and relaxed. Best of all, it only requires you, your crayons, and this book.

Some Important Considerations to Keep in Mind

Some facts about stress featured in the "Did You Know?" sections of this book are just that — *some* facts about stress, and should be regarded as such. Numerous books, scholarly works, and countless articles in the popular press are available to interested readers wanting more than an introductory and brief consideration of the topic. Our aim here is to give the reader an increased awareness of the role of stress in everyday life, and to share some techniques for stress management. In *Color Me Calm*, we emphasize coloring as *one* way to relax and perhaps add a degree of pleasure to your life even in hard times. Will coloring change your life? In a word: no. But, it is inexpensive, uncomplicated, and environmentally friendly. Activities such as coloring can bring about a positive attitude-adjustment in those willing to give it a try. We believe coloring has a calming effect for the simple reason that it works for us, and for that reason alone, we recommend it.

Keep in mind, however, that symptoms of stress can overlap those of anxiety and depression. If continued attempts to relax or reduce stress on your own are not working, or if stress is posing a threat to your health or well-being, seek professional help. Structured stress-management programs, as well as mental health counseling for anxiety and depression are widely available at hospitals and freestanding clinics around the country.

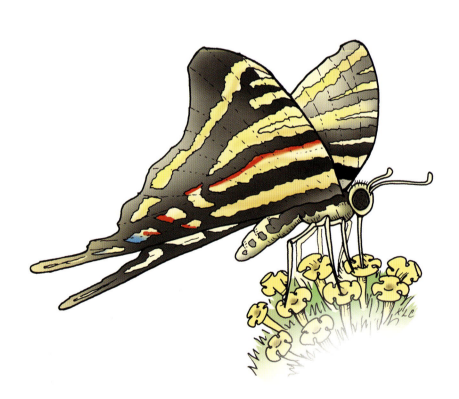

Our Thoughts on How to Use This Book

To get the most benefit from this book, use the act of coloring to change some of your attitudes and perceptions. Thoughts and emotions that seem to shade our reality can be altered by techniques that lift our spirits. The power of mood can be potent medicine.

Each plant illustration is accompanied on the facing page by the following: (a) "Did You Know?" sections — factual information about stress and stress management; (b) "Be Encouraged" sections — true stories with names changed taken from our own life experiences, along with some general observations aimed at lifting your spirits; (c) "Thought for the Day" sections — inspirational messages to help you integrate the time spent coloring into the process of relieving stress, and finally; (d) The plant description sections — selected facts about the plants for those who really do need to know the correct colors of the blooms and leaves!

While we had some progression in mind as we created this book — moving from a definition of stress to some techniques for relieving stress — each illustration with its accompanying passages on the facing page stands alone. That is, you can open the book to any page in the book and begin coloring. Or you can return to pictures you have colored in the past and re-read the text, especially the words that seem to speak to you at this particular time in your life.

The only rule when coloring pictures in the book is this. Do it your own way! Ralph Waldo Emerson said, "There are voices we hear in solitude, but they grow faint and inaudible as we enter the world." Be quiet and listen as you read and color. You can *hear* an interesting and artistic person — you — on the way to creating a masterpiece. Choose a page and begin!

Mary Virginia Graham and Madge Cloud

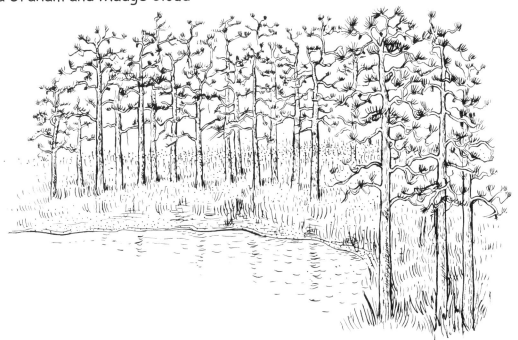

Did You Know?

What Is This Thing Called Stress? Ask friends and relatives what causes them stress and encourage them to explain how they are affected by stress, and how they manage the unpleasant feelings that stress tends to create. (Don't try this at home — unless you have lots of time on your hands *and* you are a good listener!) You will hear a variety of responses — some similar but many different, reflecting the reality that each of us experiences life in unique ways. The fundamental feature of stress is this: it is a perfectly normal part of the human condition that we all face as we adjust to our ever-changing world. And, not surprisingly, we experience *more* stress when a great deal of change occurs within a short period of time. Any definition of stress must include a consideration of *good* stress in addition to *bad* stress, or the feeling of being overwhelmed usually associated with the term *stress*. Good stress involves those exciting life experiences that leave us feeling challenged and exhilarated instead of distressed. Thus, we consider the importance of good stress in our lives in this book as well, but in less detail.

Be Encouraged

Emphasize the good things in life to help overcome negative stress. We hope that coloring becomes one of those good things for you. What a great way to get grounded: sitting quietly, crayons in hand, all attention focused on the picture before you. But before you begin coloring the illustration on the facing page, close your eyes and see yourself in the midst of this delightful hammock filled with the lovely shrub, red anise. Watch the play of the sunlight through the branches of the nearby palms. Listen to the birds calling to each other, feel the cool breeze on your face, and smell the licorice scent of the red anise. As you color, appreciate the extent to which such an activity facilitates focusing the mind and calming the spirit.

Thought for the Day

Aristotle defined happiness as the *bios theoretikos* — the solitary life of contemplation. Coloring in solitude offers me an opportunity to contemplate and reflect on how *I* would define *happiness*. Contemplation and coloring — *poetry in motion!*

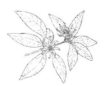

Illicium spp. or Anises. Red anise, an erect, evergreen, densely foliated shrub is one of two species of anise found in Florida, growing near woodland streams and in low, rich areas. Flowers of this anise species are deep red with numerous, ribbon-like petals, creating a bright and interesting display against the background of the dark green, elliptical-shaped, and leathery-textured leaves. Red anise is very aromatic, emitting a scent similar to that of licorice when its leaves are bruised or crushed.

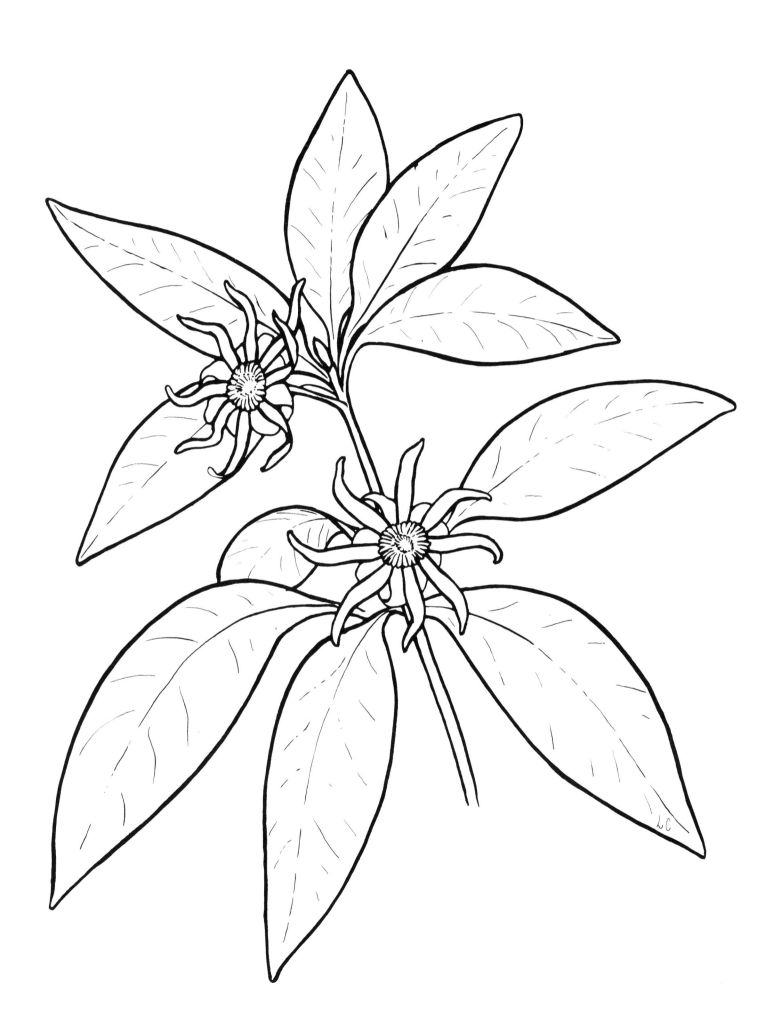

Did You Know?

Did Our Surveys and Research Yield a Definition of Stress? Well, Read On. The word *stress* is commonly used in two different ways: 1) the circumstance or situation causing us to feel unease, and 2) the physical and emotional discomfort that we experience about the situation. Stress, then, is used to denote both a cause as well as an effect, which is a little confusing. Whereas stress is neutral in quality — neither inherently good nor bad — in this book we focus on stress as a sensation of *being thrown off-balance* physically, mentally, or emotionally. This view of stress acknowledges the feelings that we often experience when demands of a situation exceed the personal and social resources we can mobilize to cope effectively and restore balance to our lives. The focal point of this book, then, is recognition and management of the unpleasant sort of stress — the kind considered synonymous with distress!

Be Encouraged

Do you remember the Carole King song that says, "You've got to wake up every morning with a smile on your face"? We can all use that as our mantra. Carole's lyrics anticipated what psychologists now say about the effect attitude has on how we live our lives. If asked to characterize a half-filled glass of water, do you say it's half-full or half-empty? If you responded *half-empty*, experts today would caution you that the *half-empty* (negative) approach is simply a *bad* habit – one that can be changed if worked on. Many dreams are within our capabilities, but if we tend to be pessimistic thinkers, we talk ourselves out of things rather than into them.

Thought for the Day

The belief that I can retrain my brain to look for joy and thus become more resilient to stress makes sense! So, how do I get started? I could begin by trying something new like coloring. That's one way to slow my life down and replace the "off-balance" feelings with "in-control" feelings. Then I can look to someone like Henry David Thoreau for inspiration: "Go confidently in the direction of your dreams. Live the life you've imagined." Can I really live the life I imagined? I want to believe that I can.

Coreopsis spp. or Tickseeds. Tickseeds are herbaceous wildflowers found in wet flatwoods and disturbed areas throughout Florida, lending beauty to otherwise dismal and drab settings. Of the 11 species of *Coreopsis* native to the state, two are especially widespread — *C. floridana* and *C. leavenworthii*. *C. leavenworthii*, featured here, has showy daisy-like flowers composed of a single layer of bright yellow rays and deep brown centers. Tall, slender but sturdy multi-stemmed stalks with sparse, slender green leaves provide ample support for the blooms.

Buckeye Butterfly. The buckeye butterfly shown here is medium-sized, overall brown in color and marked by six prominent purple-black eyespots — two on each hind wing and one on each fore wing. Buckeyes frequently get nectar from tickseeds — members of the *Asteraceae* family — a family among those favored by this species.

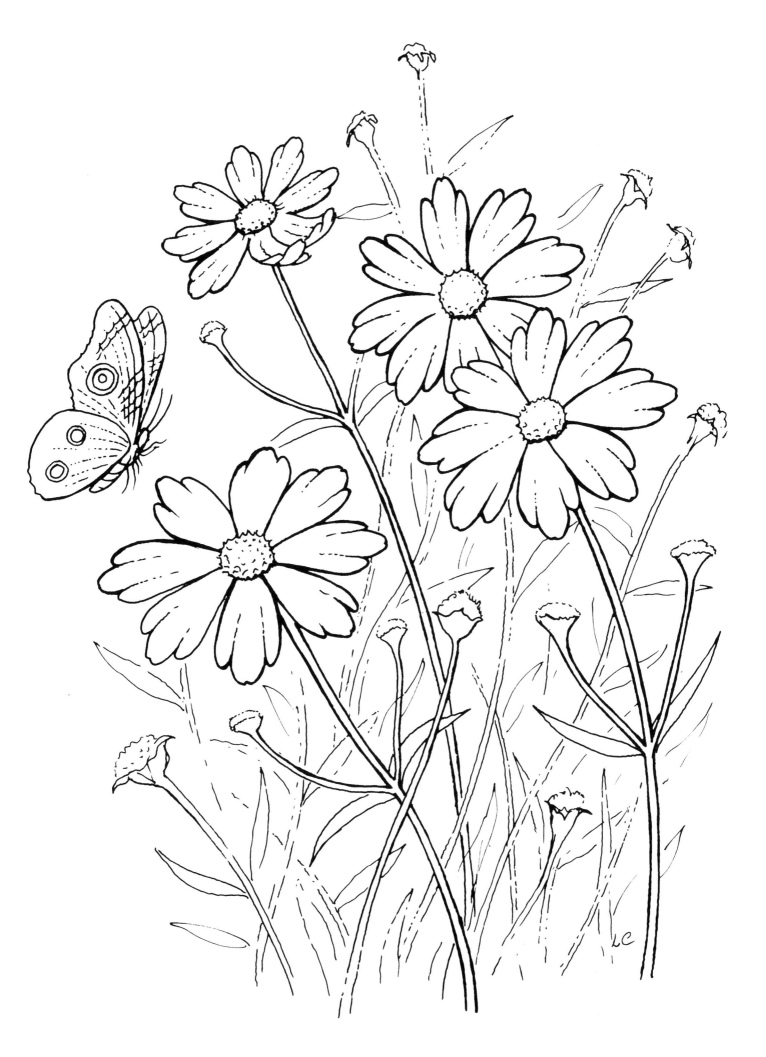

Did You Know?

Turning the Present into a Gift. Life means change, and change — for better or worse — occurs across the full lifespan. How are you coping with the stress of change? Are you living in the moment? Or do you find yourself wishing for things to be the way they were or dreaming about how much better life will be in the future, if only . . . ? Most experts agree that stress is best managed by valuing your existence in the moment through learning to appreciate whatever you *do* have. Sometimes we wait for everything to be right or settled before opening ourselves up to new experiences or new people. You may be disappointed if you rely on fate or chance to make changes in your life. Instead, be proactive. Seek out beneficial interests or pursuits, especially during the difficult times when the temptation is great to be passive and withdrawn. The very act of taking action to develop positive attitudes can, in and of itself, improve one's mood. Things don't necessarily happen for the best, but it is possible to make the best of things that happen.

Be Encouraged

We all can benefit from developing personal portfolios of stress-coping strategies such as regular physical activity, meditation, social support, and some forms of relaxation that work for us. Blogging, e-mailing, texting, tweeting, and Facebooking are staples of life for many. With so much to do, to know, and to learn, however, there is a real risk of becoming overwhelmed by a virtual flood of information. At some point, you may ask yourself, "Am I improving my life or wasting my time?" Years ago, Sid, a poet friend of mine (MVG) proposed a twist on the famous *Rolling Stones'* lyric: "You can't always get what you want; you get what you *need*." Sid's take was this: "You can't always get what you want; you get what you *can*." I remember thinking initially that he was just plain cynical. Over the years, I finally understood what Sid was saying, and I recognized the authentic meaning of the phrase *getting what you can*. Far from being cynical, getting what you *can* from life is really about wanting what you already have rather than always needing that elusive *something else*. Are you getting what you *can* from life?

Thought for the Day

Walt Whitman writes in *Leaves of Grass*: "Happiness is not in another place, but in this place . . . not for another hour . . . but this hour." Whitman, with these words, is telling me — albeit in a much more elegant way — to follow Sid's advice: "Get what you *can*. Now!"

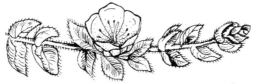

Kalmia hirsuta or Hairy Wicky. Hairy wicky is a small, hardy shrub closely related to mountain laurel with a native range in Florida that extends southward in the peninsula to about the upper third of the state. Found in pine flatwoods and wetlands, this upright shrub is distinctive for its numerous stems and evergreen leaves covered with stiff hair-like projections. (The Latin term *hirsuta* refers to these characteristic projections.) The small bell-shaped flowers, pink to pale purple in color, are arranged in clusters of two or three. Leaves are opposite, small, oval to elliptic in shape, dark green in color, and have almost no stalk.

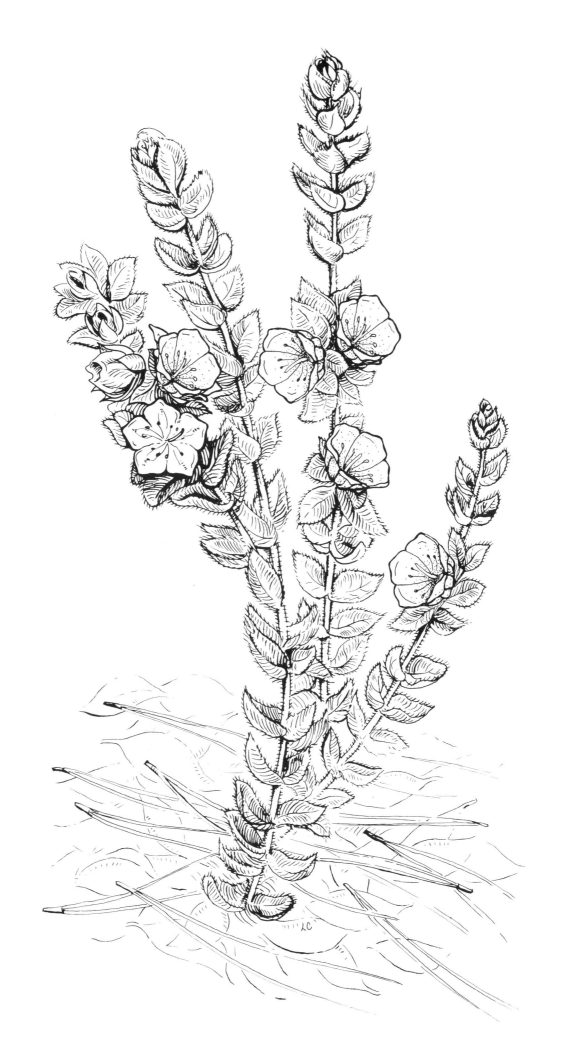

Did You Know?

Should I Stay or Should I Go? When the brain senses a threat, it automatically activates the "fight-or-flight" response — called the alarm reaction — prompting several physical changes preparing for survival of a potential threat. The alarm reaction makes it possible to react in ways that boost ability to fend off physical threats. In most modern life situations, however, we are much more likely to face symbolic threats or threats to our emotional well-being rather than physical ones that the fight-or-flight response was designed to manage. The stress response hasn't changed much over time even though most situations that produce stress in today's world are such that neither fight nor flight is a practical solution.

Be Encouraged

Did you see the movie *Avatar*? Now there was some stress — physical *and* emotional. I (MC) don't like to admit that I was a little leery of seeing a movie in 3-D because I had read that many people get nauseated or dizzy by that third dimension, and being the dizzy dame I am, I thought I was a prime candidate. I lived to tell the tale — it is a spectacular movie. Imagine humans — visiting another planetary system — transformed into avatars of these remarkable indigenous peoples, the Na'vi, and learning to ride dragon-like creatures — pretty scary even from the audience seats. And these same human avatars try to save the Na'vi from being annihilated by the mercenaries hired by the corporation conducting the mining operations. See this movie for another dimension in dealing with physical and mental stress, because just as there are many different responses to stress, there are also abundant ways of managing its effects — positive courses of action that don't involve ignoring or glossing over the problem (and rarely require riding a dragon!).

Thought for the Day

Each day, I will look for — and find — at least one good moment, however small. Time spent coloring gives me the opportunity to be reflective. In the words of our *first* First Lady, Martha Washington, "I am determined to be cheerful and happy, in whatever situation I may be; for I have also learned from experience that the greater part of our happiness or misery depends upon our dispositions, and not upon our circumstances."

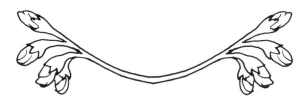

Trichostema dichotomum or Forked Bluecurls. This small dainty wildflower is a member of the *Lamiaceae* or mint family, and is found growing in dry, sandy, open sites along roadsides in north central and coastal Florida. Flowers are two-lipped, blue in color and appear at the tips of short branches arising along the leaf axis. Long, curled stamens characterize this airy and elegant little plant. Leaves are green, lance-shaped, and opposite in arrangement, providing a lacy and charming background for the blooms.

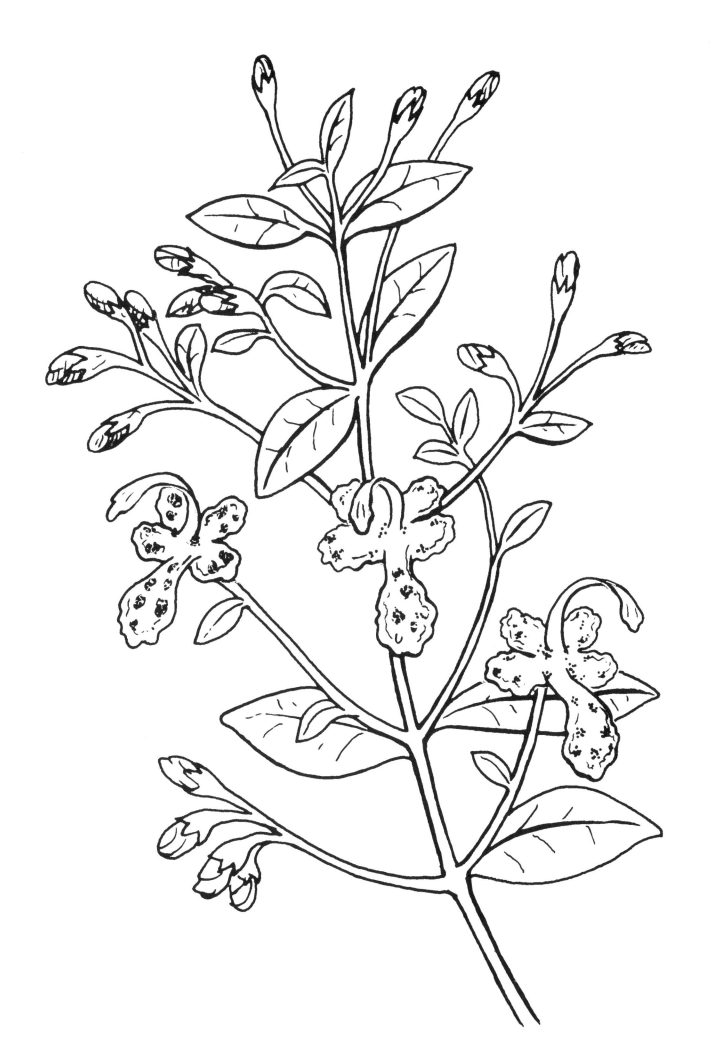

Did You Know?

Physiology of the Stress Response: A Close-Up Look at the Mind-Body Continuum at Work. In times of stress, the alarm reaction signals a number of structures within the brain to go on alert. The hypothalamus, amygdala, and pituitary gland instantaneously exchange information with one another and dispatch signaling hormones and nerve impulses to the rest of the body, mobilizing a cascade of interrelated physiological events aimed at optimizing survival. Adrenal glands react to the alarm by releasing epinephrine (adrenaline), inducing elevations in heart rate, breathing, and blood pressure — all of which work in concert to deliver oxygen faster throughout the body to maximize strength and stamina. Adrenal glands also release glucocorticoids — in humans, the relevant glucocorticoid is cortisol — to fuel an energy boost. Nerve cells release norepinephrine — a neurotransmitter closely related to epinephrine — that tenses the muscles and sharpens the senses to prepare for action. Digestion shuts down as the blood supply is diverted to the brain and muscles where it is most needed. *Note to self: This is no time to eat that chocolate cupcake!*

Be Encouraged

Take time out of your busy day for some leisure activity — it's beneficial! We love doing crossword puzzles and sudoku — just concentrating on something outside ourselves for a few minutes; but amazingly, we love coloring even more. We never hang a completed crossword puzzle or sudoku on our refrigerators, nor do we go back and look at them at some later time — nope — we're done with them. But we both enjoy our coloring enough to either display, return to look at later, or share what we've colored with each other. Coloring can make your mind feel refreshed and better able to deal with life's demands. Right now, head for "Destination Calm." You won't find it on any map, but you can find it by coloring if you let yourself go.

Thought for the Day

I am going to "let go" and enjoy coloring. "People don't stop playing because they grow old; they grow old 'cause they stop playing." ~ Ziggy Marley. Why not give myself time to play? I definitely don't want to grow old!

Gaillardia pulchella or Blanket Flower. This colorful herbaceous wildflower with a native range throughout Florida often grows in difficult habitats such as sandy roadsides, medians, and parking lots. Brightly colored daisy-like flowers feature reddish to maroon rays, tipped in yellow. The central disk is deep purple, providing a splendid contrast to the surrounding rays. Leaves are alternate, lance-shaped, hairy and bright green on this slender stalked plant. Numerous members of the *Asteraceae* family grow in Florida — only the blanket flower, however, features the unique two-toned red and yellow flowers.

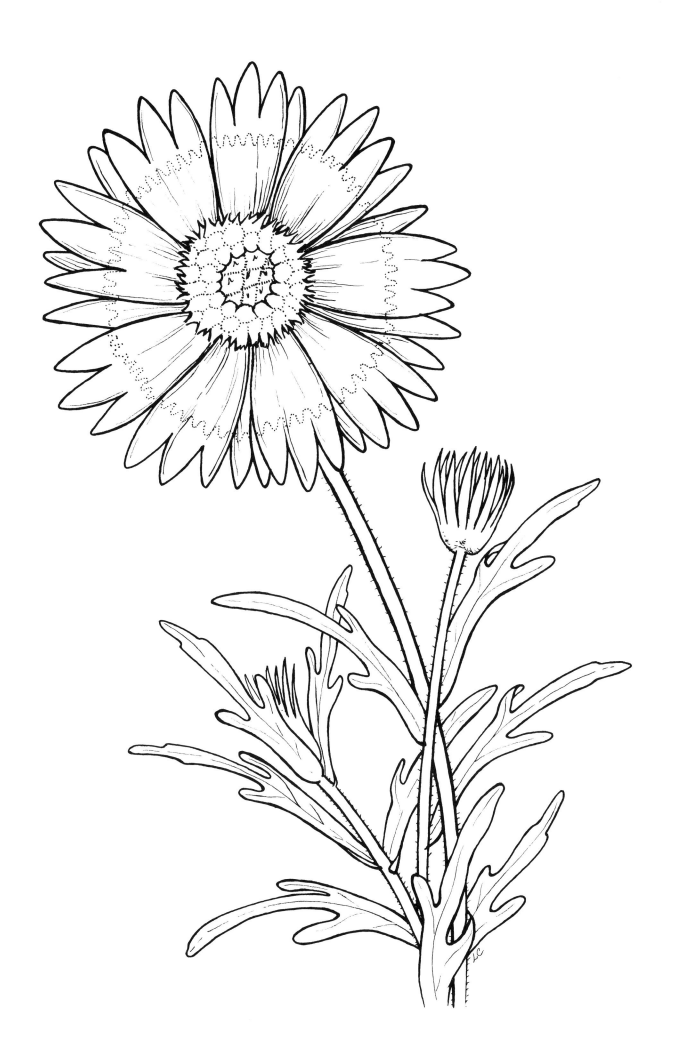

Did You Know?

Would Someone Turn That Alarm Off? Because our brain continues to interpret all threats as equally harmful, a confrontation with our boss is likely to feel as threatening to modern man as an encounter with a wild boar was to prehistoric man. Who knows? In some cases, it just may be! Our body requires a high level of energy expenditure to initiate and maintain the stress response. Once we feel our jaws clinch and our stomach tighten, we know it's time to counter the fight-or-flight response and restore equilibrium. Continuation of this phase over a prolonged period of time in response to perceived or actual threats is neither practical nor useful. When the threat passes, hormone levels return to normal. If, however, danger in the form of acute stress comes too often, or if stress becomes chronic, damage to the body — both mental and physical — can occur.

Be Encouraged

When my (MC) granddaughter, J., was in fourth grade, she went on a field trip into the city. Her assigned seatmate deserted her and joined two other little girls on the seat behind her. She later described to me how the three of them laughed at her, teased her, and generally tried to make her life miserable. "But Gram, I just looked out the window and pretended I didn't hear them. I wouldn't let them get *in* (I think she meant *under*) my skin." That a nine year old had such a mature attitude in dealing with a really stressful situation has never ceased to amaze me. To restructure your *own* thinking about stress, try this moment-by-moment approach when you feel overcome by emotions. Regroup by taking a mental step back to figure out what should be done first, and bring your full attention to doing it. Once the first action is taken, take a slow, deep breath. Decide what comes next and move on to it.

Thought for the Day

The more practical skills I acquire to manage stress, the better prepared I am to really appreciate life. Much the same as J. in the story above, I won't let things "get in my skin." Instead, like J., I will think pleasant thoughts — she wisely chose looking out the train window at the ever-changing landscape as a way to stay calm and maintain her composure. My solution is to spend a few minutes coloring — it's easy, practical and calming. One of the most courageous women in history, Eleanor Roosevelt, used these words to describe growth that comes from dealing with stressful life situations: "You gain strength, courage, and confidence by every experience in which you really stop to look fear in the face . . . you must do the thing you cannot do."

Gelsemium sempervirens or Carolina Jessamine. This sparsely to densely foliated multi-stemmed, twining, evergreen vine is found in hammocks and flatwoods, southward to central Florida, and is often used in landscaping to conceal fences and similar structures. Flowers are bright yellow, fragrant, and trumpet-shaped. Leaves are dark green, shiny, lance-shaped and arranged in an opposite pattern on the vine. The twining habit and fast growth patterns along with attractiveness to both butterflies and hummingbirds make this vine an excellent choice for many landscaping needs. The buckeye butterfly shown here is described on a previous page — see the tickseed illustration.

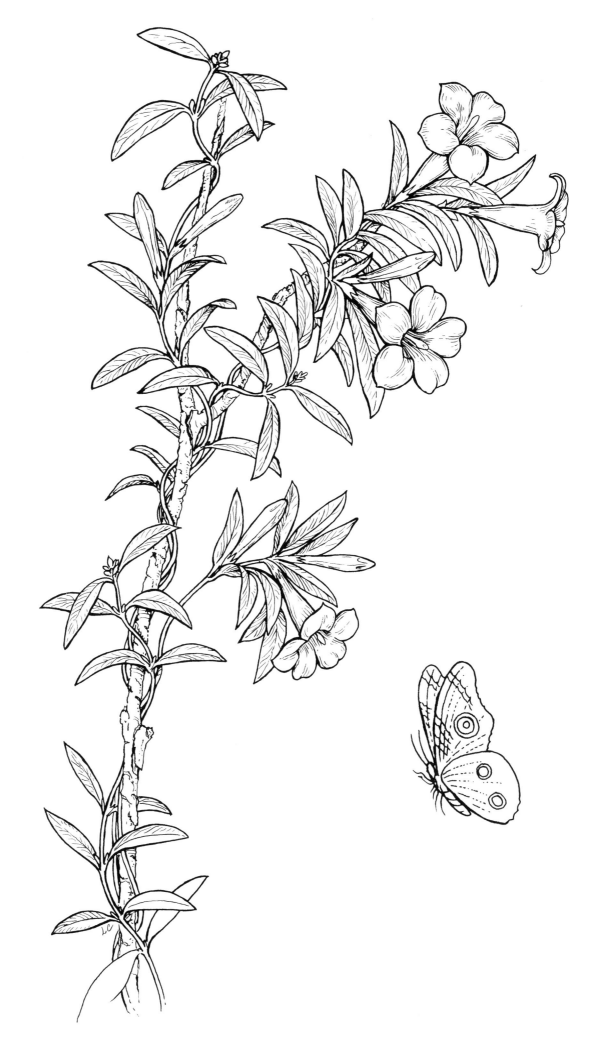

Did You Know?

Acute Stress: Usually Less Cute Than It Sounds. Stress comes in two forms — acute and chronic — and each has unique features and health consequences. *Acute* stress is prompted by a specific event and is usually short-lived. For example, you are late for an important appointment; your teenage son is involved in a fender-bender that is sure to make your car insurance rates skyrocket; you accidentally delete an important file at work and can't figure out how to retrieve it — you know the scenarios that are part of the daily grind for most of us. However, when a person's life is filled with frequent episodes of acute stress — that is, their life is a study in chaos and crisis — epinephrine and norepinephrine levels are elevated repeatedly possibly causing damage to the cardiovascular system, increasing the risk of coronary heart disease and stroke.

Be Encouraged

Faced with a situation that is acutely stressful, the first order of business is to regain your composure and equilibrium. Once the shock subsides from the initial jolt you feel when the reality of a situation hits home, detach yourself emotionally from what has happened as best you can, and concentrate on breathing deeply and rhythmically. Breathe S-L-O-W-L-Y. Controlled breathing lowers your heart rate and helps focus your attention. This allows your thoughts to stop racing and the spinning out of control sensations to wane. Here's one technique to try. Take three slow, deep breaths, breathing in through your nose, and out through your mouth, making sure your belly — not your chest — is rising and falling. Your belly should swell on the in-breath and flatten on the out-breath, while your chest remains still with both inspiration and expiration. Now, start coloring, belly-breathe, have fun and get calm.

Thought for the Day

In times of stress when the pressures of the world are too much, I can find calmness by being quiet, closing my eyes, and creating for myself a peaceful place removed from the jarring rhythms of modern life. Controlled breathing helps me experience greater self-awareness. For a few minutes, I can color in solitude, away from the discordant beeps, rings, hums, chatter, and buzzes that drown out the beautiful sounds of silence.

Hydrangea quercifolia or Oakleaf Hydrangea. This large upright deciduous, irregularly branching shrub is found on bluffs and ravine slopes in central peninsular Florida. Several features — flowers, leaves, and bark — contribute to its beauty. Blooms are grouped in large showy clusters appearing in spring and persisting in various stages until late fall — transitioning in color from white to creamy white, to pinkish to purplish, and finally to light brown. Large leaves — about 8 inches at maturity — are equally showy: opposite in pattern, dark green on the upper surface, lighter green to whitish on the under surface, and ovate in overall outline with 3 to 7 deeply lobed and toothed edges. Bark is similarly attractive — medium brown in color and exfoliating in strips over time to expose lighter inner bark. Altogether, this is one of Florida's most ornamental native shrubs.

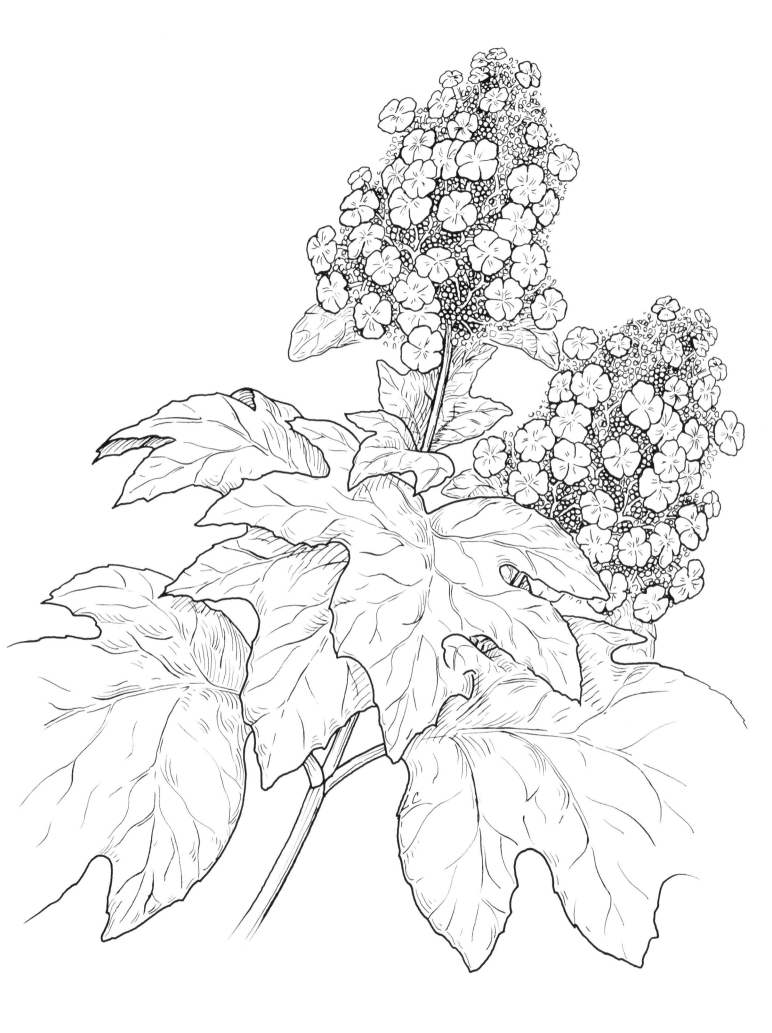

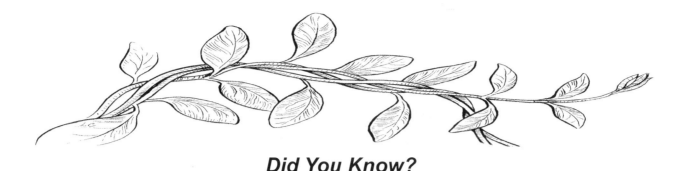

Did You Know?

Chronic Stress: I Can't Get No Satisfaction. Events or situations that occur over a prolonged period of time that you find distressing — even if others consider them inconsequential — can cause *chronic* stress. Chronic stress can also be precipitated by major life events — death of a loved one, divorce, a move to a new location and a new life — all events considered stressful to most people. Those experiencing chronic stress may feel that there are no outlets for frustration, no sense of control, and little hope that something better will follow. The impact of chronic stress on health can be substantial, with adverse effects differing from those of acute, episodic stress. Whereas acute stress is likely to target the cardiovascular system, chronic low-level stress stimulates a persistent secretion of glucocorticoid hormones, primarily cortisol. Higher than optimal levels of these hormones are known to cause impairment of the immune system, loss of bone mass, and memory problems. Left unchecked and untreated, both acute and chronic stress can exert a generalized wear and tear on the body, making us feel old before our time.

Be Encouraged

Let us share with you two stories about *chronic* stress. One of our relatives — an uncle — spent 15 years caring for his wife who has Alzheimer's disease. He often said, "I'm tough. I'm an ex-Marine and I can take it." Well, he did take it — 24/7 for 15 years. He wouldn't let anyone help him, but now that his wife is in a nursing home, he himself is so debilitated that he needs help! Now the second story concerns another relative who is a Hospice volunteer. He sits with terminal patients while their caregivers take time off. And that is why he does it — to help the caregivers. He has told us so many stories about how grateful these people are to him for helping them to maintain their own perspective, health, and even sanity! Many of us are sometimes reluctant to turn to others in time of need, but when we do allow others to help us, they feel "needed," and we both benefit. Mutual interdependence is a reality of life, so let's make use of it.

Thought for the Day

When was the last time I let someone do some small favor for me? So often, I say, "NO," to any offer of help, sometimes before I even take time to consider it. I'm so independent that I find myself having to multitask all day long just to stay one step ahead. But I'm going to change that. For the next few minutes while I color, I will quiet my thoughts and take delight in the present before it slips always. I will enjoy the experience fully, remembering the words of John Lennon: "Life is what happens while you are busy making other plans."

Lonicera sempervirens or Coral Honeysuckle. This twining, climbing vine can be found in the rich hammocks, sandhills, and open woodlands of central Florida, and is an excellent vine for fences, arbors, and trellises. The trumpet-shaped flowers are a dazzling deep orange to scarlet red in color. Leaves are opposite, oval to oblong in shape, and dark green in color, providing a delightful background for the colorful blooms. The ruby-throated hummingbird shown here is described on a later page — see the trumpet creeper illustration.

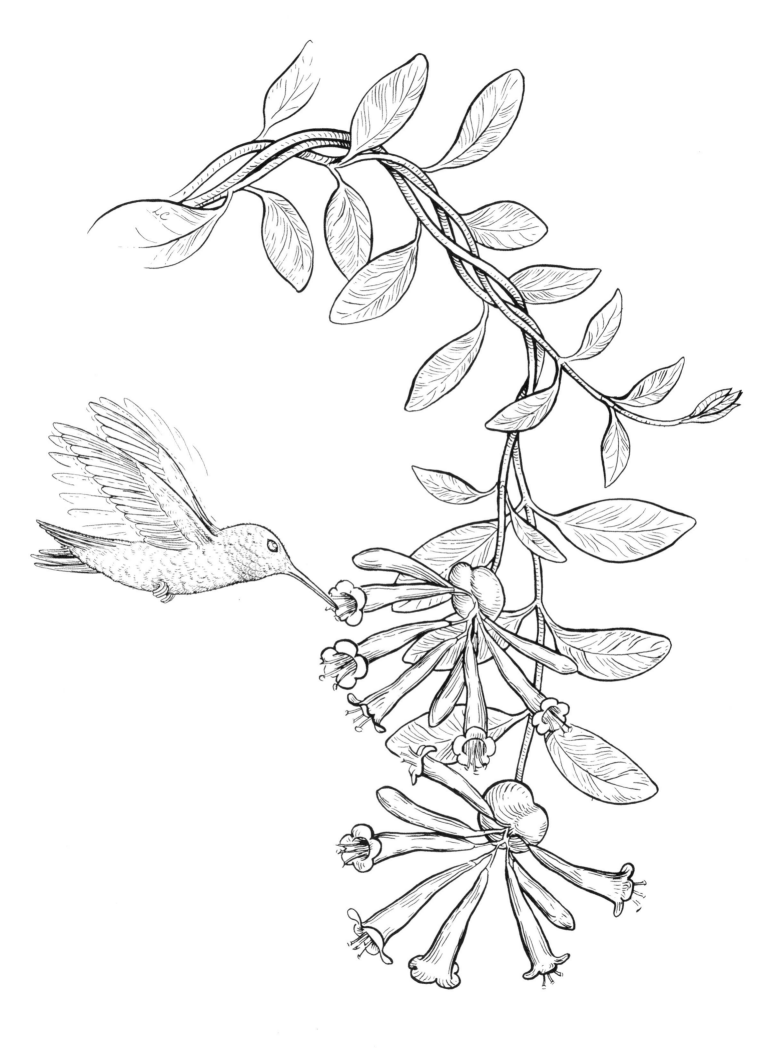

Did You Know?

Should I Be Afraid or Excited: Is That a Real Vampire or the Actor from the Twilight Movie? Activation of the stress response is not necessarily linked to the degree of danger faced by the individual. For example, such everyday experiences as having a misunderstanding with a friend or family member or being stopped for speeding can initiate release of stress hormones that trigger the fight-or-flight response. But some elements of the alarm reaction — a heightened degree of concentration and increased energy levels — can help in many instances. For example, mobilization of these physiological changes can be advantageous to someone racing against a deadline or preparing for an important meeting or function. On the other hand, helping turns into hurting when these stress-induced physical changes are triggered to levels out of proportion to the actual situation, or when the stress response continues unchecked for too long.

Be Encouraged

We think you would agree that getting a divorce often triggers *unhelpful* stress. Barb, a recent divorcée, had this to say about her experience: "Some days I feel as though I'm broken into a thousand pieces. Other days, I feel as though I will make it. I do know that every day that passes helps me grow stronger." Another cliché — *Time heals all wounds* — but one that continues to ring true. We hope that you use this book and the coloring as a way to stay centered when things are chaotic. Coloring can give you a sense of calm that lasts for hours, and you and others will notice and appreciate the attitude change.

Thought for the Day

How good am I at recognizing which stress is helpful and which is harmful? Do I make time for myself every day — a calming time that gives me space to be objective about how I'm choosing to live my life? Is it time to make a fresh start? As I move forward, I will forget the lost opportunities in my life and remember the words of Alexander Graham Bell: "When one door closes another door opens; but we are often looking so long and so regretfully upon the closed door, that we do not see the ones which open for us."

Rhododendron austrinum or Florida Flame Azalea. This deciduous upright leggy shrub has a native range that includes slopes, bluffs, and wooded stream banks in the Florida panhandle and in the north central part of the state. Flowers are tubular, yellow to orange in color and sweetly fragrant. The showy clusters of blooms are grouped near the tips of branches. Leaves on this multi-stemmed shrub are alternate, bright green in color and widest at the tip.

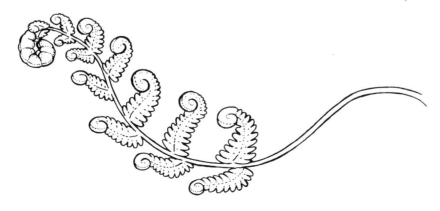

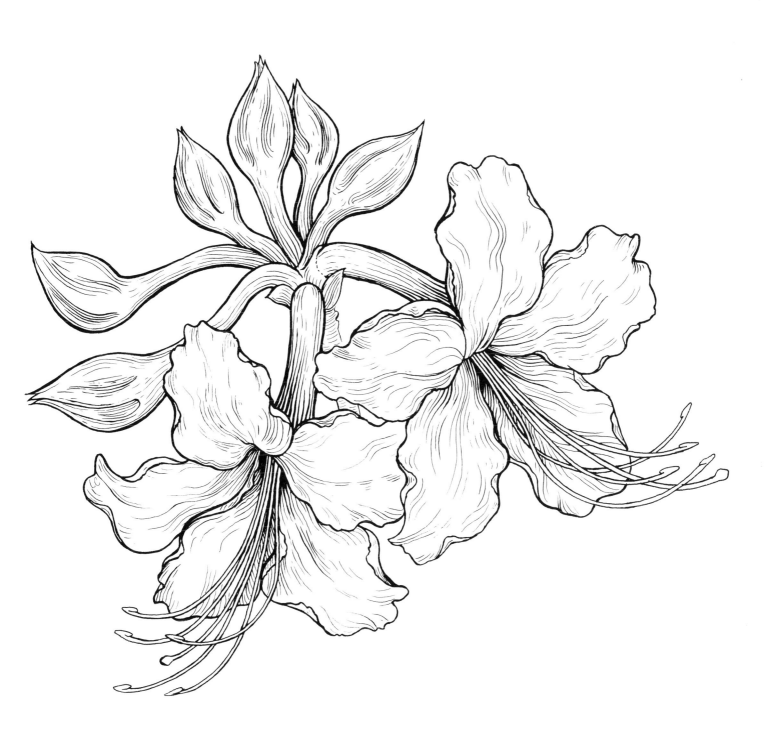

Did You Know?

Stress Is Like the Swiss — Neutral. Any sort of change has the potential to make us feel stressed, even change for the better. Thus, change itself is less important than how we view the change. The old adage, "One man's meat is another man's poison," pretty much sums it up. To illustrate, retiring from work may be experienced very differently by those involved in this life transition — some may feel totally lost, while others feel that they have finally found themselves. Emotional and physical responses are highly personal and individual processes — not surprising, since we are each unique.

Be Encouraged

Stress challenged Abraham Lincoln throughout his life: his mother died when he was just a young boy; his father wanted him to work rather than get an education; his first love, Ann Rutledge, died; he was president during the Civil War — one of the most horrific wars in history. Lincoln is often portrayed as having a melancholy disposition and as having suffered from depression. One modern scholar, Joshua Shenck, has proposed that Lincoln developed his famous story-telling prowess as his way of coping with stress and melancholy. He further argues that, "Lincoln didn't do great work because he solved the problem of his melancholy. The problem of melancholy was all the more fuel for the fire of his great work." You don't have to be a Lincoln to find ways to rise above the problems that life throws at you.

Thought for the Day

Coloring this lovely hibiscus blossom allows me to symbolically grow a flower in my life and to view change as opportunity. Abraham Lincoln expressed the deliberate and kindly way he dealt with people and events in these words: "I always plucked a thistle and planted a flower where I thought a flower would grow."

Hibiscus coccineus or Scarlet Hibiscus: This upright, sprawling, slender shrubby herbaceous perennial is found on the edges of wetlands and swamps as well as along roadsides in north and central Florida. Large brilliant red 5-petaled, cup-shaped blossoms open over a period of several months in the spring and summer. Leaves are dark green and divided palmately (like an open palm with fingers extended) into 3 to 7 deeply narrow, pointed serrated lobes, providing a unique background for the crimson flowers. Many plants in the *Malvaceae* family — of which the scarlet hibiscus is a member — serve as host to a variety of larval and adult butterfly species.

Gray Hairstreak and Common Checkered Skipper Butterflies: At the top of the illustration, is a gray hairstreak — blue-gray, with each fore wing marked by a relatively straight post-median line that is white, bordered on the inside edge with a narrow orange line. At the bottom is the common checkered skipper — also blue gray in color (female is black) — with both sexes featuring large white spots forming median bands across each fore wing and each hind wing.

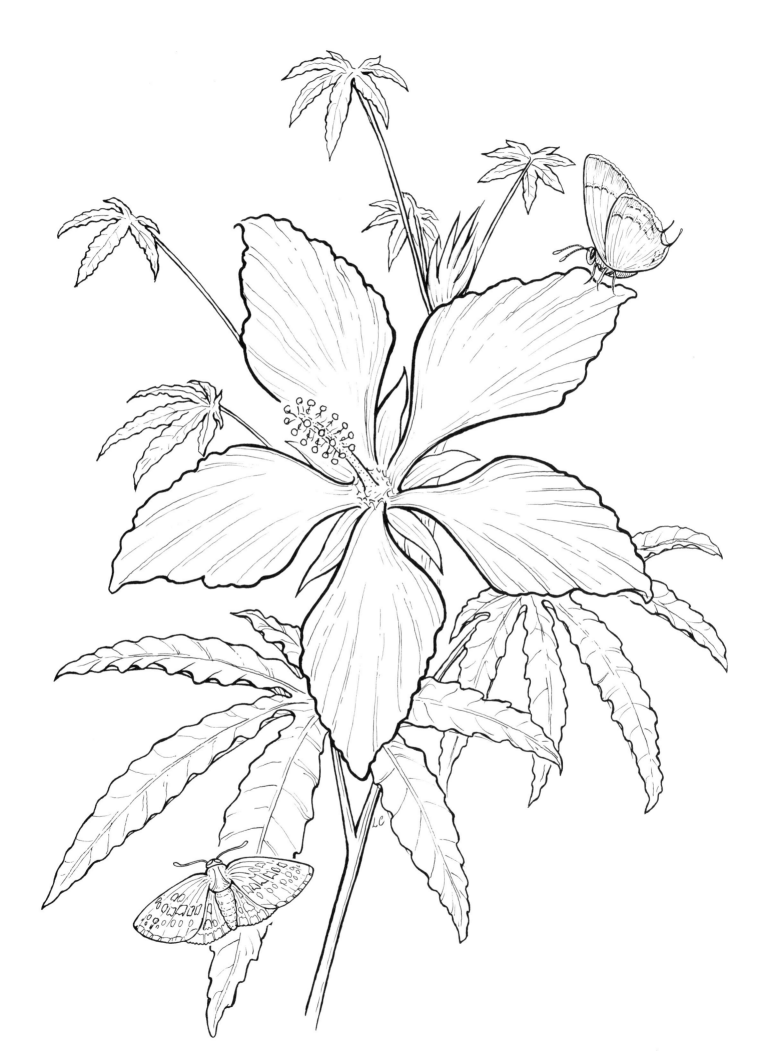

Did You Know?

Am I Finally Pickin' Up Those Good Vibrations Just Like the Beach Boys Promised? Feelings of stress let us know that something is different, and in some cases, *not right*. Viewed from this perspective then, stress can supply the motivation we need to take action to restore a sense of equilibrium or balance. For example, the stress of preparing for the role of leading lady in a local community theatre production can inspire a burst of creativity that turns an ordinary performance into a truly dazzling one! Handled correctly, then, the unpleasant feeling of stress can be an early warning system that helps us get prepared — enabling us to change a situation, if necessary, or alter our response toward something we cannot change.

Be Encouraged

Our ninety-year-old mother has lived alone for over thirty years. She is hard of hearing, has chronic back pain, suffers an occasional bout of depression, and is sometimes fearful in her ever-changing neighborhood. This same woman gardens, rakes leaves, makes fabulous pies, does needlework, and drives herself to church every Sunday. We say she does so well because she always tries to live up to those "shoulds and oughts" in her head. But when we hear her praying aloud in her bed at night, we know she has something even more going for her! Mother's system works for her, but the good news is that each of us can learn to control our stressors regardless of the personal and situational factors that we bring to any situation in our lives.

Thought for the Day

How am I doing with handling my stressors? Am I aware of the early warnings my mind and body send me when I am in a stressful situation? I will use those warnings to remind me to create a positive response. Maybe I will "whistle a happy tune," or meditate, or think of a new way to see the problem; but right now, I am going to color this picture. Coloring was fun when I was a kid, and it's fun now. Thank goodness some things never change! How can I apply this to my life? By remembering the words of Marcel Proust: "The voyage of discovery lies not in finding new landscapes, but in having new eyes."

***Asimina* spp. or Pawpaws**. At least three species of *Asimina* are found in Florida in various habitats from coastal dunes and sandhills to mesic woodlands. The species featured here, *A. triloba*, or common pawpaw, has rather inconspicuous flowers, dull red in color, hanging below the oval-shaped leaves that are alternate and medium to dark green in color. Attractiveness and desirability of this plant are enhanced by the fact that the common pawpaw — along with all of plants in the *Asimina* spp. — is larval food of the zebra swallowtail butterfly.

Zebra Swallowtail Caterpillar. Shown here is a zebra swallowtail caterpillar or larva, yellow-green in color with black and yellow stripes. This caterpillar emits an unpleasant odor that helps fend off predators.

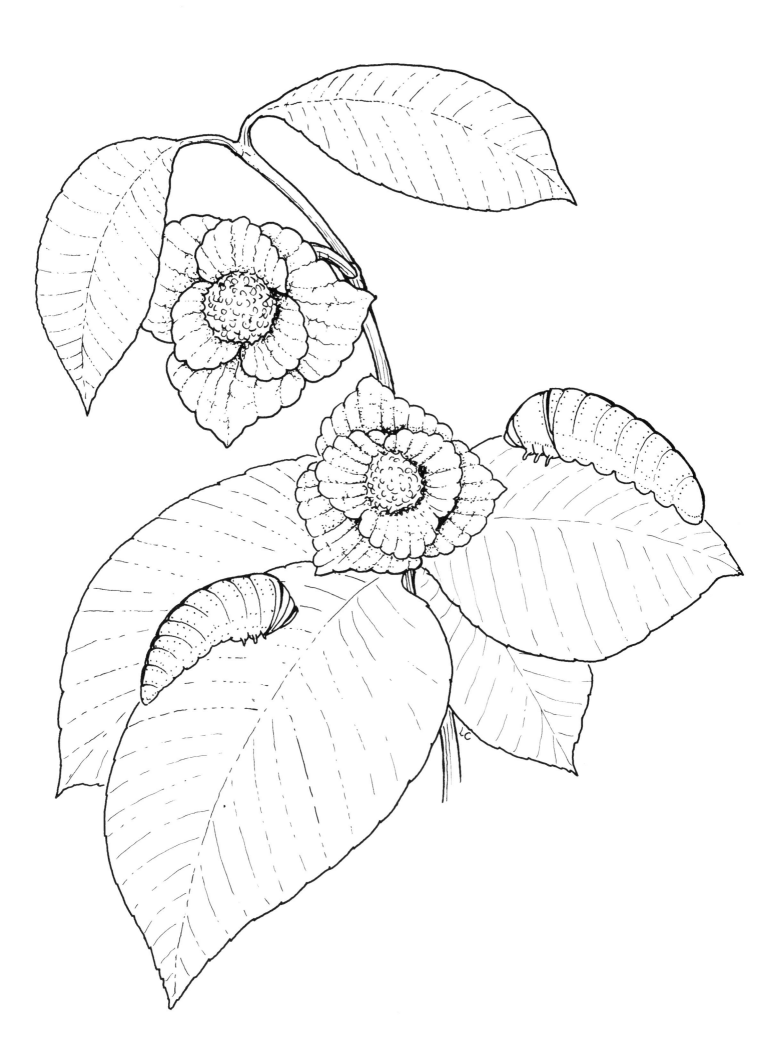

Did You Know?

Bless This Stress? Avoiding stress completely is not possible in today's world, nor is it desirable. In fact, life would be very dull without some stress, don't you agree? Cheering on our child or grandchild in a close soccer or tennis match can be exhilaratingly stressful, and most of us wouldn't miss the chance to experience *that* stress for the world! What is crucial, then, is learning to manage one's response to unpleasant stress, the kind of stress that seems to occur all too often in many of our lives.

Be Encouraged

The honest recognition that there are some things in our lives that we are simply powerless to change — acceptance — is not the same as recognition of defeat. Acceptance means that we are willing to face a certainty in our lives without bitterness or blaming. When my family and I (MC) moved from a small town to a city of several million, my friend Vicky wanted to know how I was coping. I could only respond, "Some mornings I wake up with a primal scream!" Just facing the commute to my job on crowded, unfamiliar expressways was enough to make me want to stay in bed. And of course it was the rainiest season in the history of the city, so this country girl was literally up to her hubcaps in flooded viaducts all too often. To be honest, all I could do was to keep putting one foot in front of another and accept that my life had changed. Acceptance is not easy, but it's a reality we all have to face.

Thought for the Day

"In the depth of winter I finally learned that there was in me an invincible summer." ~ Albert Camus. And believe me (MC), the winters in Chicago can reach some real depths!

Campsis radicans or Trumpet Creeper. This high-soaring, aggressively colonizing woody vine climbs by aerial rootlets, and can be found in a wide variety of woodlands across much of the panhandle and central peninsular regions of Florida. Flowers are fiery, deep orange-red, broadly trumpet-shaped, waxy in appearance and up to 3 inches long. Leaflets are dark green on the upper surface, lighter on the lower, and are ovate shaped with coarse teeth and an elongated tip.

Ruby-Throated Hummingbird. Dazzling flowers of this vine never fail to attract ruby-throated hummingbirds — eastern North America's sole breeding hummingbird — one of which is pictured here. These small hummingbirds with their slender, slightly downcurved bill and rather short wings glitter like jewels with bright emerald or golden-green coloration on the back and crown, contrasting elegantly with their gray-white underparts. Males have a brilliant, iridescent or rainbow-colored red throat most evident in bright light or full sun. These tiny birds fly straight and fast, but can stop instantly, hover, and, with great precision, adjust their position to facilitate feeding from their preferred nectar sources. By early fall, they're bound for Central America, with many crossing the Gulf of Mexico in a single flight!

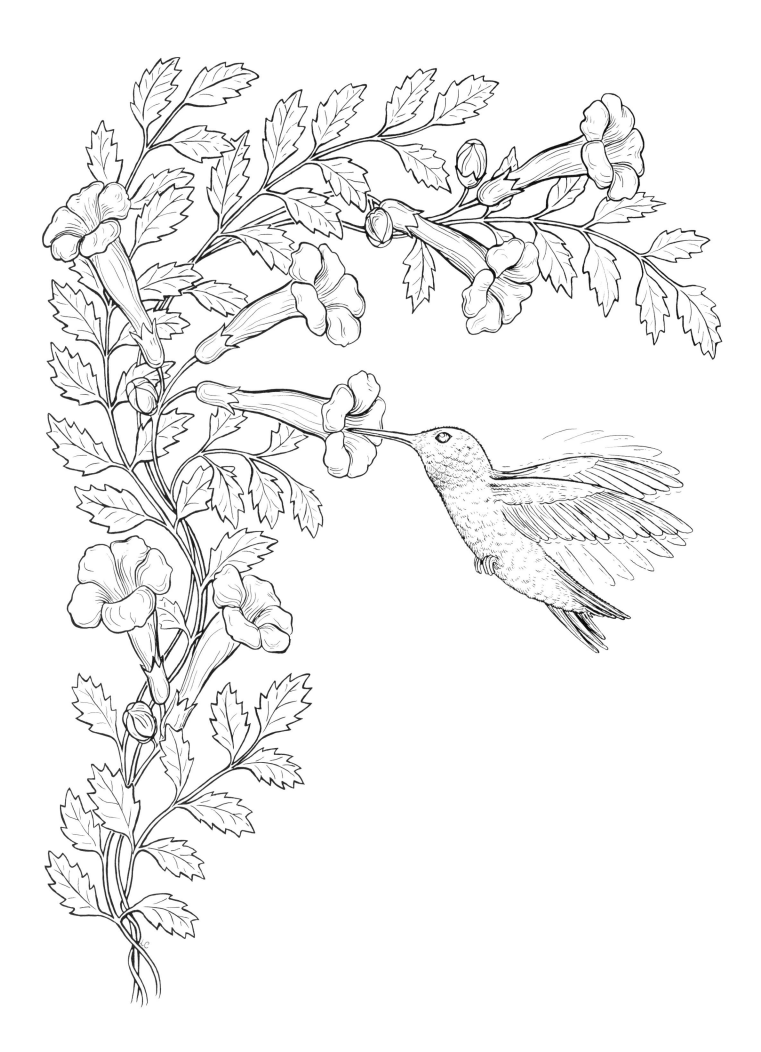

Did You Know?

Stop the World I Want to Get Off! Maybe Not, What I Really Want Is to Feel Better. In a recent poll relating to stress among persons living in the US, almost one-third of responders believed that negative stress was significant in their lives, adversely impacting their health. Interestingly, when they were asked about their most frequently used coping mechanisms to counter stress, a substantial number of people reported using alcohol and overeating in order to feel better. Obviously, both of these lifestyle choices do little to manage stress; instead, they further impair health. Fortunately, there are many positive behaviors that can both prevent stress as well as help us quickly recover from feeling *stressed-out*. Such behaviors are collectively known as the *relaxation response*, a response that can induce physiological changes including reduced heart rate and blood pressure, decreased muscle tension, and slowing of brain waves. Do you believe that the stress in your life is adversely affecting your health? How do you deal with stress?

Be Encouraged

Just as there are many different responses to stress, there are also abundant ways of managing its effects — positive courses of action that don't involve burying one's head in the sand. While it may seem like common sense to let go of our feelings of stress, don't we often find ourselves with a sense of dread or uncertainty? I (MC) sometimes wake up in the middle of the night with that feeling, and I have to sort through why I'm feeling that way. I'm relieved when I actually find something concrete that is triggering the feelings so that I can *consciously* work on it. And if it is just a vague feeling or something I can't change, I can *consciously* let it go.

Thought for the Day

Today, I am going to sit down and color, even though my inner critic wants me to spend time remembering all the petty annoyances of the day. Choosing to rid my mind of negative thoughts and gaining clarity by engaging in a pleasant activity — coloring — is a productive way to spend a few minutes and a smart move toward a life full of positive thinking. When I give time to my own improvement, I find myself relaxing. My spirits are lifted, and when I move back into my busy world, I can better cope with it.

Salvia coccinea or Tropical Sage. This tall, erect, and colorful perennial wildflower can be found nearly throughout Florida, thriving in hammocks, disturbed sites and sandy woodlands. Whorls of bright red flowers are borne in conspicuous, showy spikes. Leaves are green, opposite, oval in shape and notched along the margins.

Bombus or Bumblebee. Shown here are bumblebees, important pollinators of wildflowers and members of the bee genus *Bombus* — containing more than 250 known species — in the family *Apidae*. The species featured here has black and yellow body hairs, arranged in bands. The soft nature of the hair, called pile, gives them a "fuzzy" appearance. Like their relatives, honeybees, bumblebees feed on nectar and gather pollen to feed their young, making them important pollinators of wildflowers.

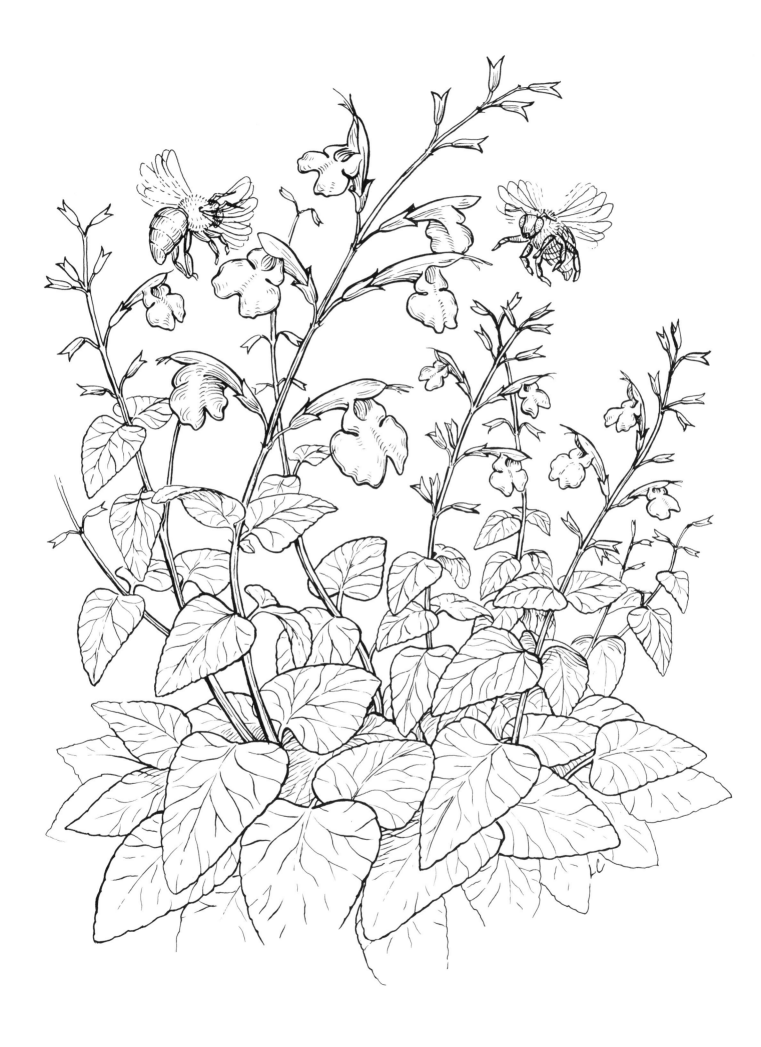

Did You Know?

Yes, We Can! All of Us, Even Me. The last couple of years have been really rough for pretty much everyone. In times like these, people often react by becoming more easily frustrated, anxious, and depressed. Stressed out individuals have a really easy time seeing all the negatives in both self and others. On the other hand, when we train ourselves to notice the good things around us, we widen our perspective and are more likely to find options and solutions that elude us in our negative state. Positive thoughts help us lock in an optimistic outlook on life — and there is a direct correlation between what we expect from life and what really happens. Recently, the US Army contracted with researchers to develop strategies to teach soldiers skills for becoming more resilient to the stresses of military service, highlighting the fact that it is possible to cultivate positive emotions, even in adulthood.

Be Encouraged

Sometimes all we need to do is change the tape that runs in our heads — the one that engages in catastrophic thinking by saying things like, "Oh, this is terrible!" in situations that really aren't so bad in the whole scheme of things. Reframing a stressful situation, or putting it into perspective as something that can be coped with rather than something that is overpowering, can reduce the intensity of emotional reactions to stress. At other times, the best approach may be to recognize that some situations simply can't be changed, no matter how much we wish otherwise. In the movie *Lake City*, Sissy Spacek plays a mother who has accidentally killed her son. She has many other problems as well, and the way she copes with them is to decide which ones she needs to let go of. She writes out on a piece of paper those that she can't do anything about and lets them fly away on the wind. Anyone can use this technique. This is a great symbolic act to signal that we have consciously let go of something that we cannot change.

Thought for the Day

I want my outlook on life to be based on realistic optimism, and I will continue to develop techniques for achieving this goal. Right now, I will write down one stressor that I need to let go of and toss it out! Then I will color, relax, and think about Anne Frank, who even as she was forced to live in hiding to escape the Nazis, wrote, "I don't think of all the misery but of the beauty that still remains." I too will look for that beauty — fixing what I can in my life and letting the rest go.

Rhexia mariana or Pale Meadowbeauty. This perennial wildflower is a member of the *Melastomataceae* family, with 3000 species including herbs, trees, and shrubs. *Rhexia*, featured here, is found in meadows, marshes, and bogs throughout Florida. Flowers — white or rose-colored to purple — are composed of four petals attached to a cylindrical floral tube. A central cluster of ornate, yellow-orange stamens provides a foil to the understated simplicity of the elegant petals. Slender, lightly hairy stems support attractive dark green leaves that are opposite, densely hairy and lance-shaped.

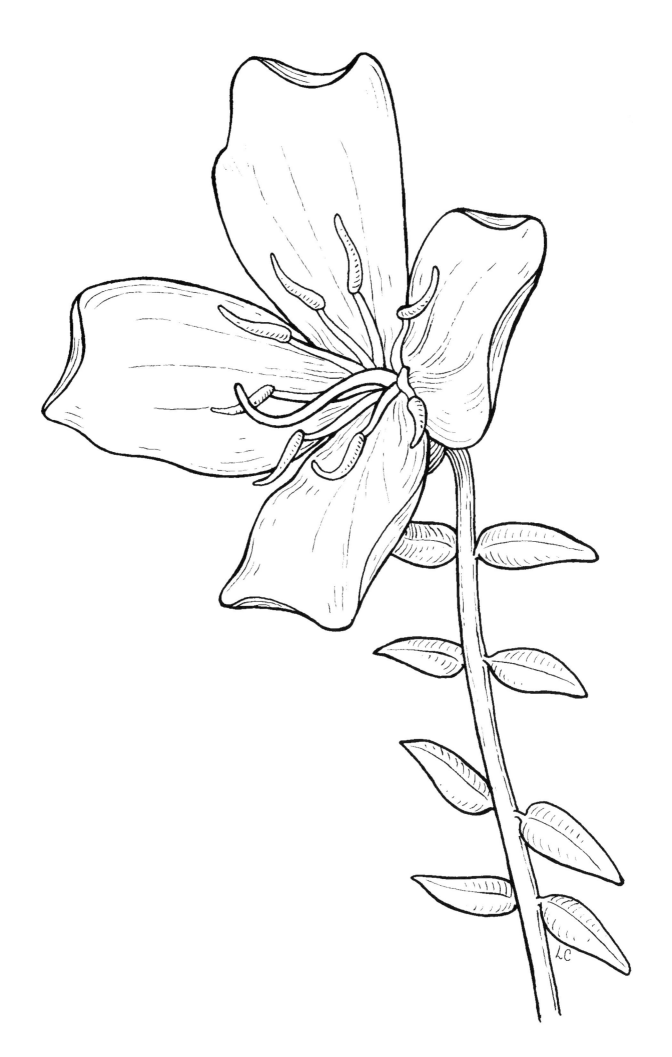

Did you Know?

Dopamine: The Main Currency of the Pleasure Pathway — And Unrelated to Feeling Like Dopey, the Most Endearing of Snow White's Seven Dwarfs. The scientific tie between good feelings and good decisions is called the "dopamine hypothesis." When we are in a good mood, parts of the brain that have dopamine receptors — regions responsible for thinking and working memory — are activated. There is strong evidence to support the theory that positive affect helps us make better decisions and enables us to find innovative answers to perplexing problems.

Be Encouraged

Have you ever noticed how animals are able to adjust to the natural flow of their lives? Two years ago, my (MVG) 12-year-old cat, Pinkie jumped from the car behind the veterinarian's office — I had failed to securely lock the door on the pet carrier. Immediately, he dashed into a nearby wooded area, and the more I chased, the faster he ran, quickly disappearing into the woods. Over the next few days, I combed those woods, talked to strangers, put up "Lost Cat" signs, placed ads in the newspaper, and did everything else I could think of to find Pinkie. When not searching, I was in bed, crying my eyes out and feeling guilty. "Cats who run away from home usually come back," a woman I encountered on my search told me, trying to give me hope. "But he didn't run away from home," I lamented. "I let him out of the car just half a block from a 6 lane highway which he'll have to cross and then *walk for a mile and a half* to get home!" My story has a happy ending. Somehow Pinkie managed to muster the courage, determination, and strength to find his way home, arriving on Thanksgiving night. His mile and a half journey took 6 days — his white coat was matted, his small pink paws, scratched and dirty, and he was thinner than before. He let himself in through the cat door. My son heard the little click of the door, and exclaimed, "Pinkie is home!" even before Pinkie himself walked into the room and headed straight over to be petted.

Thought for the Day

Pinkie's story is about acceptance of life as it is, with its sometimes frustrating, sometimes painful realities. Today, I will take one moment to value my existence — dwelling neither on the pain of the past nor the fear of the future, recalling the words of Albert Camus: "If there is a sin against life, it consists perhaps not so much in despairing of life as in hoping for another life and in eluding the implacable grandeur of this life." With these graceful words, Camus is saying to me "Don't let the perfect be the enemy of the good."

Ruellia caroliniensis or Wild Petunia. Wild petunia is one of at least five species of *Ruellia* native to Florida. This unbranched, 2-3 foot perennial wildflower is found on roadsides, in disturbed areas, and sandhills. Blooms cluster near the top of the short hairy stems and are light purple in color with a slender corolla tube and five petal-like lobes. Leaves are dark green, opposite in arrangement, and ovate in shape.

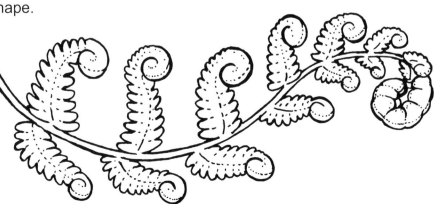

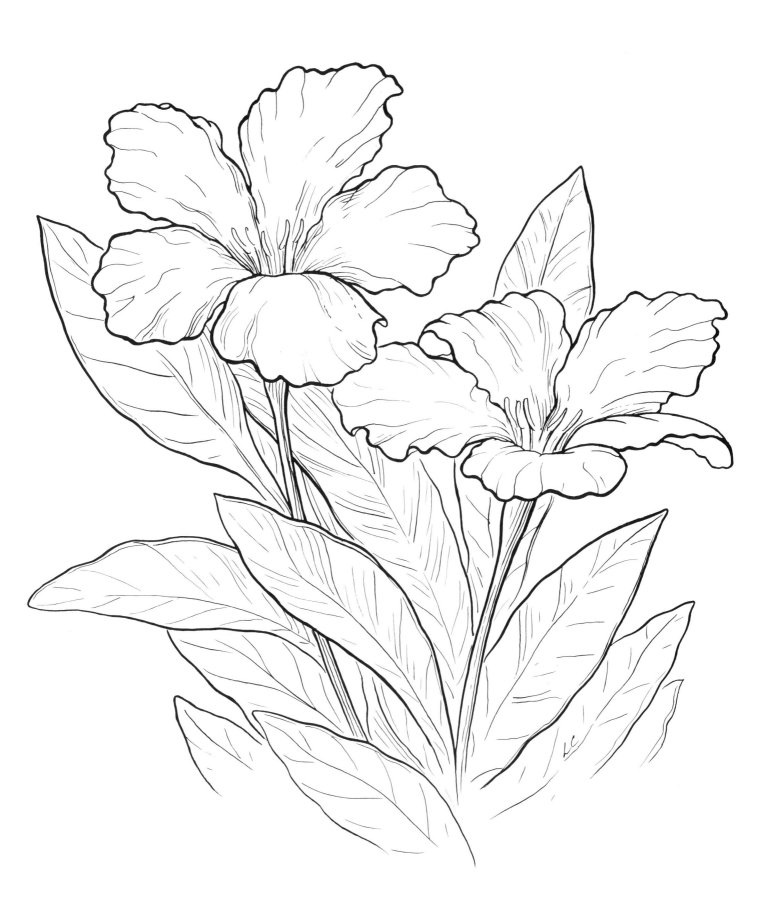

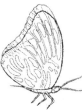

Did You Know?

Doing the Same Thing Over and Over and Expecting A Different Result? Maybe It's Time to Try Something New. Just as stimulating an area of the hypothalamus in the brain can initiate the stress response, relaxation in some form can reverse the impact of stress and counter its harmful effects. Ours is the loudest, noisiest century ever. Isn't it ironic that in such a harsh, discordant environment, we tend to erect barriers between ourselves and solitude? Somehow, escaping inharmonious noise and seeking silence is frowned upon. In fact, engaging in quiet time can be viewed as the *awake* version of sleeping — it has very therapeutic benefits on multiple body systems.

Be Encouraged

The notion that every hour must be spent "productively" seems to be part of our cultural conditioning. Anything we can do to relax our minds and bodies on a regular basis, however, enhances our ability to successfully manage stress. We King sisters are really not all that caught up in online chatting, tweeting, texting, or Facebooking. We readily admit that it could even relieve stress for some, but since we aren't that "into" it, we were quite relieved to read that the human brain can only sustain about 150 meaningful friendships at any given time (and that seems rather high to us — no doubt because neither one of us feels capable of sustaining that many!) There are ways, maybe Facebooking included, to restore serenity even in the midst of a stressful day. Coloring — which we "Sour Grapes" endorse — can elicit a "relaxation response." You may have a hard time accepting this, but silence really is golden!

Thought for the Day

One way to turn off the noise in my mind is to be silent and to color. "If women were convinced that a day off or an hour of solitude was a reasonable ambition, they would find a way of attaining it. As it is, they feel so unjustified in their demand that they rarely make the attempt." ~ Anne Morrow Lindbergh. I will attempt every day to find that hour of solitude, consciously controlling what I allow into my mind.

Passiflora spp. or Passionflower. Passionflowers are hardy, flat-lying or climbing, spreading deciduous vines featuring dazzling, ornate flowers with a native range of open hammocks, roadsides, fencerows, and disturbed sites. *Passiflora incarnata* — the more common, widespread and showy of the two species of *Passiflora* found throughout Florida — is featured here. Blooms are large, solitary pale to dark lavender, very intricate and ornate, with two outer rings of filamentous or fringed coronas surrounding conspicuous stalked ovaries and stamens. Large, alternate dark green, deeply three-lobed leaves provide a fitting background for the lavender flowers. Passionflowers are a larval food plant for zebra longwing and gulf fritillary butterflies.

Adult Gulf Fritillary. Shown here is an adult gulf fritillary, a medium-sized bright orange butterfly with black markings on each dorsal fore wing surface. The ventral hind wings have numerous large silvery spots, framed in black.

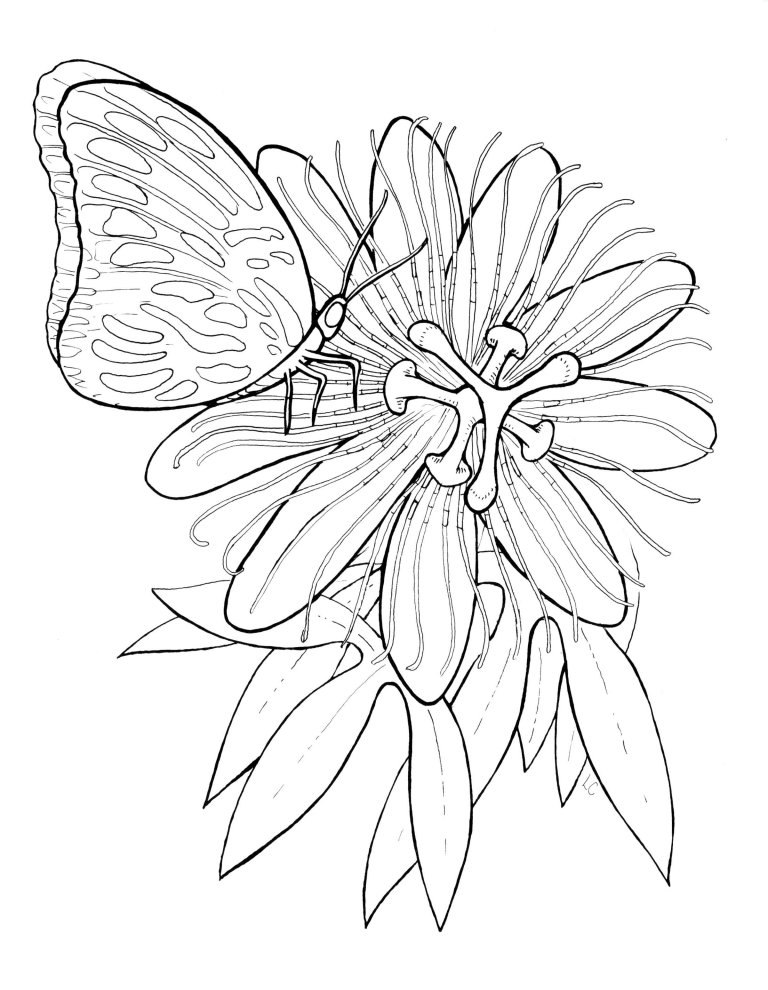

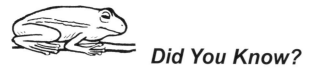

Did You Know?

Goodbye, Hello Dollies (The Cookies, Not the Musical)! How do you comfort yourself when you feel stressed-out? Be honest! Do you manage the stress or does it manage you? Authorities agree that consistent use of thoughtful and purposeful stress management techniques empowers us to make better lifestyle choices throughout the day. We are less likely to use alcohol, tobacco, feel *too tired* to exercise, or consume sugar-laden, high-calorie, nutritionally-poor foods when our stress levels are low. One way to keep our stress levels low is to train ourselves to use some of the techniques we have talked about earlier — take a deep breath or two, slow down and seek solitude, think of the good things in our lives, get perspective (things are often not as bad as they seem), and let it go when necessary. And, by all means, reach for those color crayons!

Be Encouraged

"Emphasizing a positive approach to stress" may sound contradictory, but we found out it's possible when our friend Lucy who was being treated for lymphoma shared her "F" words with us. She obviously didn't mean the usual "F" word — no, her words were "Faith, Family, and Friends." Lucy was divorced, had two children, and was now having bone-marrow transplants to treat the lymphoma, but she always believed she would overcome this disease and live to see her children become adults. Her "F" words have kept her going for over ten years and counting.

Thought for the Day

I will create my own paradigm for coping with stress. I know how to do it, so today as I color, I will reflect on my resiliency and search out ways that I can be the best person I can be for myself and for those whom I love. I understand that character is not determined by events in my life. Rather, my response to events — both good and bad — ultimately reveals my character to myself and to others.

Erythrina herbacea or Cherokee Bean. This spiked, sometimes climbing, herbaceous to woody multi-stemmed shrub, unique among Florida's native shrubs is found in dry, open woods and along sandy roadsides. The bright red flowers of this shrub are very narrow and long, borne in distinct upright spikes. The dark green leaves are equally attractive with a pronounced three-parted triangular shape and pointed tip.

American Green Tree Frog. Featured here is an American green tree frog, a medium-sized amphibian, colored in shades ranging from bright yellowish olive to intense lime. Kermit the Frog of *Sesame Street* fame was modeled after this charming little frog with its smooth skin and large toe pads. At night, this common backyard species can be seen at porch lights, searching for insects. During the day, they may be found resting on plants near floodplain sloughs.

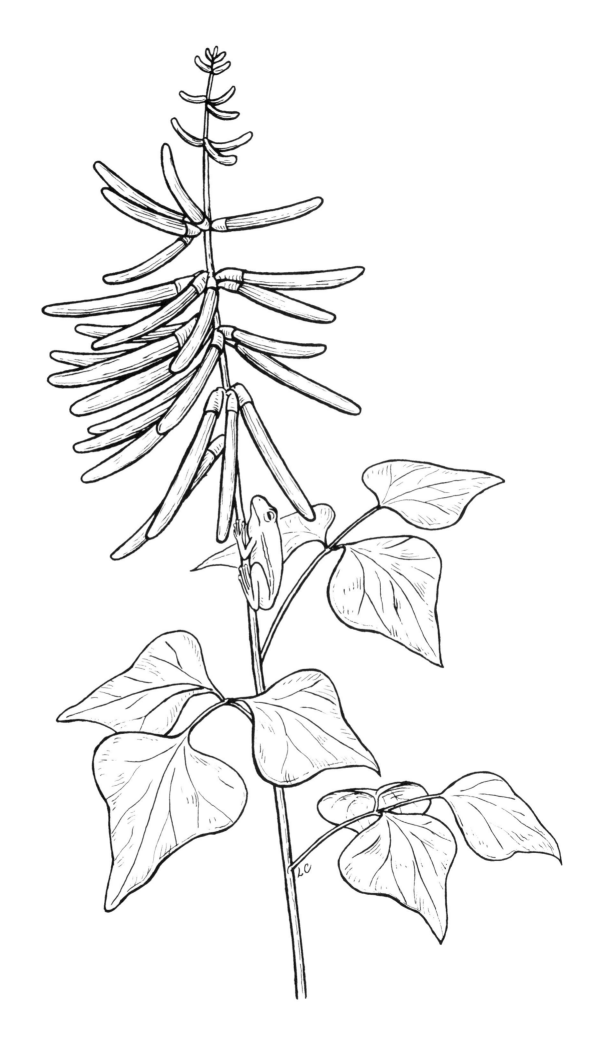

Did You Know?

Come On! Everybody's Doing It — Or Should Be. Play is not just for children — it has a valuable role in helping us develop cognitive skills of creativity, logic, and problem-solving. Further, play allows us to put the rest of the world on *pause* and encourages us to smile and forget our problems for a while. There is more than one path to a happy and fulfilling life — you may find your path more easily when you take time to savor each day.

Be Encouraged

"Resilient people enjoy themselves like children do. They wonder about things, experiment and laugh," writes Dr. Al Siebert in *The Resiliency Advantage*. You'll recall that we created this coloring book because we were *playing* with our grandchildren. We hope that you have found some information and relaxation from reading and coloring that will enhance your life, and that you will continue to find time to play!

Thought for the Day

Today, I celebrate that I am ready and eager to try something new — coloring. I will happily engage in an activity that people generally associate with children, and will laugh good-naturedly if I am teased and called *weird* for coloring. Paul McCartney's take on *weird* is a bit convoluted, but it gets the point across: "I used to think that anyone doing anything weird was weird. I suddenly realized that anyone doing anything weird wasn't weird at all, and it was the people saying they were weird that were weird." Well, obviously, I am not "weird" for coloring, and I do know I am definitely on my way to becoming a new, improved, UN-DISTRESSED ME!

Hymenocallis latifolia or Spider Lily. This elegant clump-forming perennial wildflower has a native range of coastal dunes and swales (shallow troughs between ridges), mangrove thickets, open rocky sites, beaches, and flatwoods of central Florida. The white, fragrant flowers have 6 narrow petals surrounding a funnel-like center and 6 elongated stamens tipped with showy yellow anthers (pollen-bearing structures in the stamen). The dark green glossy leaves appear strap-like, arising from the plant base in a dense, erect to arching clump, providing a pleasing background for the flowers.

Lobelia cardinalis or Cardinal Flower. This erect perennial wildflower is found in flood plain forests and edges of streams in central Florida. Showy, red flowers in terminal spikes resembling flaming spires are arranged singly along a common elongated unbranched axis. Erect, leafy stems, often in clusters, hold green lance-shaped leaves.

Peninsula Cooter. Shown here is a peninsula or Florida cooter (*Pseudemys floridana*), a turtle species commonly found in slow-moving streams and still bodies of water with soft bottoms and aquatic vegetation in the Florida peninsula as well as in the panhandle. Active year-round, the species spends most of the day basking on logs. The top of the shell (carapace) of the peninsula cooter is uniformly dark green with a pattern of parallel yellow markings stretching out toward the sides. Coloring and markings of the head and legs are similar to that of the carapace.

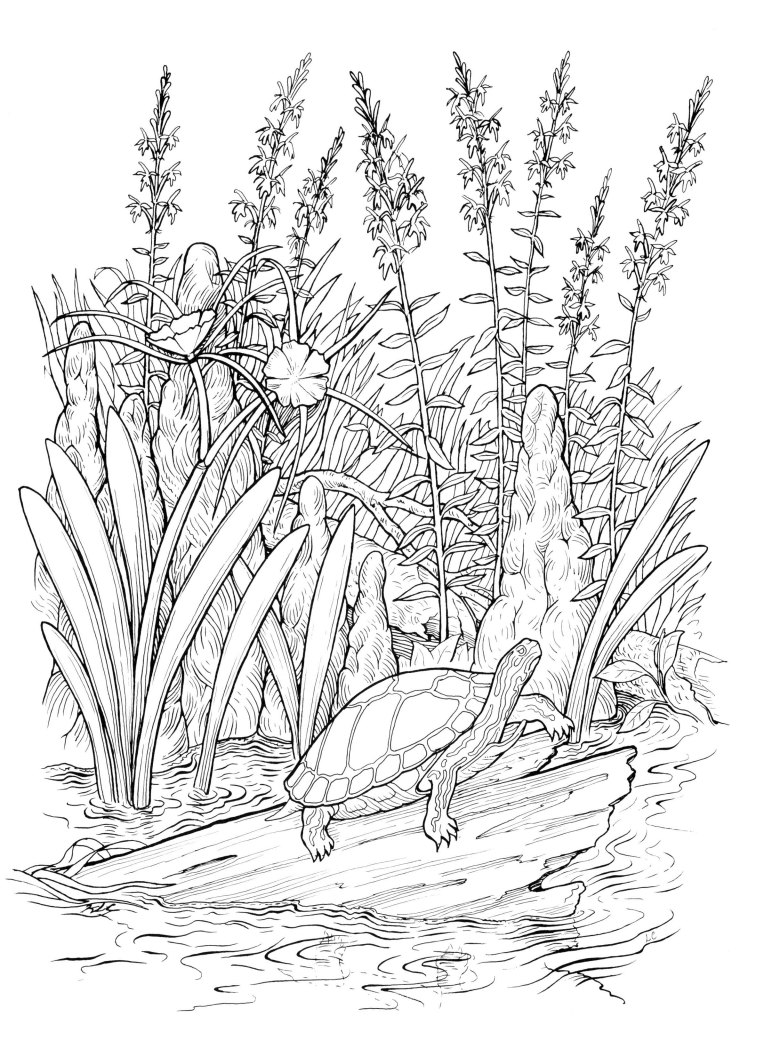

About the Authors

The King sisters — Madge Cloud and Mary Virginia Graham — were born and raised in Helena, located in the Arkansas Delta. They were educated by the wonderful *Sisters of Charity of Nazareth** at Sacred Heart Academy, a small school housed in a beautiful and historic pre-Civil War building. The community, and indeed the entire state of Arkansas, suffered a great loss when the school closed and the building was demolished in the 1960s.

Madge received a Bachelor of Arts degree from Illinois State University and a Master's degree in English Literature from Northern Illinois University. She writes plays for a book reviewer in the Chicago area.

Mary Virginia received Bachelor and Master's degrees in nursing from the University of Florida, and a PhD in nursing from the University of Texas at Austin. She has taught nursing as well as practiced as a registered nurse and nurse practitioner, and is coauthor of a series of books for nurse practitioners. She has a special interest in the consequences of stress on mental and physical health.

*Of special note, the *Sisters of Charity of Nazareth* are one of 21 women religious congregations featured in an exhibit — **Women & Spirit** — appearing at various venues throughout the US in 2010-2011, beginning at the Smithsonian in Washington, DC. The exhibit celebrates the contribution of Catholic Sisters in health care, social justice, and education. On display is a handwritten note by Abraham Lincoln, dated January 17, 1865, aimed at protecting the lives and property of the *Sisters of Charity of Nazareth* during the Civil War.

About the Illustrator

Louis Clark has had a lifelong interest in art as applied to scientific and biological subjects. He received a Bachelor of Arts in Art from the University of Florida and a Master of Science in Medical Illustration from the Medical College of Georgia. His website is www.bio-graphix.com.

Sources for Plant Descriptions

Lady Bird Johnson Wildflower Center. The University of Texas at Austin. Available at www.wildflower.org, accessed December 1, 2009.

Nelson, Gil. (2003). *Florida's Best Native Landscape Plants*. University Press of Florida, Gainesville, FL.

Plant Atlas. Available at www.plantatlas.usf.edu, accessed December 1, 2009.

In Loving Memory

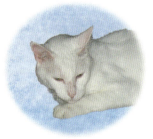

Pinkie, beloved cat of the Graham Family, whose story appears in this book, died in March 2010, shortly before the book was completed. We miss him very much.

Color Me Calm: Stress Management Through Coloring Featuring Florida Native Plants

Ordering Information

You may use the order form below or visit our web site at **www.colormecalm.com** to place an order.

Make check or money order payable to *Color Me Calm*.

Order Form

Name:_____

Street:_____

City:_____ State/Zip Code:_____

Price: $14.95 each (+ 6.75% sales tax for Florida residents, total = $15.96)
(**Note:** There is no charge for mailing orders to our customers who live in the continental US.)

Substantial price reductions are available for orders of 10 or more books. For details, please e-mail mvgraham@yahoo.com.

Fax order: *(352) 378-1441*

Mail order address:
Color Me Calm
5127 NW 62nd Street
Gainesville, FL 32653

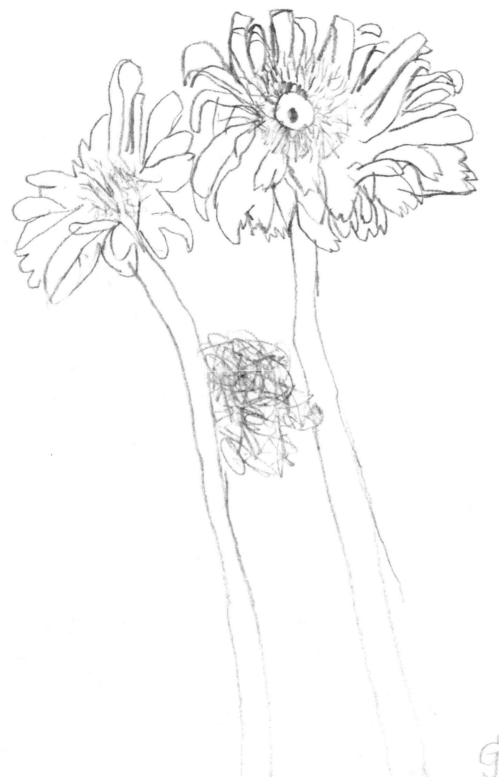